First Aid at Sea

This book provides rapidly accessible guidelines for dealing with medical emergencies in a small boat or yacht at sea. It is not a comprehensive textbook on first aid and it is strongly recommended that all seafarers should receive general training in first aid. Responsibility for first aid should be given to a nominated and appropriately trained member of any crew. The environment of the vessel and the sea imposes major limitations upon what can be achieved in the care of illness or injury while afloat. First aid treatment that may be appropriate ashore has to be modified at sea.

The aims of *First Aid at Sea* are to:
- preserve life
- prevent further harm
- relieve pain and suffering and
- deliver a live patient ashore.

Safety and simplicity should guide the management of every case so that any unnecessary treatment or intervention is avoided. Conditions that threaten life or limb demand heroic action and conditions that threaten permanent damage or disability require urgent attention. Many other conditions will be infinitely better treated ashore even after a significant delay, and all that is required at sea is basic damage limitation and pain relief.

Seek help early in all cases of serious illness or injury, and for other cases if any doubt exists about correct management. Before using the radio, write down details of the case as listed on page 31.

Keep this book in a readily accessible place so that it is instantly available.

> While every attempt has been made to present safe and effective first aid guidelines in this book, the authors and the publishers do not accept any responsibility for the outcome of any first aid or treatment that is administered to any person in any circumstance whatsoever.

The recommendations for Basic Life Support (BLS) are based on the 2015 Resuscitation Guidelines (Resuscitation Council UK). These have been modified in response to Covid-19. For the latest information see: www.resus.org.uk.

The Covid-19 pandemic has created additional health challenges for sailors. It is essential that sailors are aware of, and comply with, the national guidelines that apply wherever they are sailing. A country can refuse entry on health grounds. Quarantine can be enforced at the cost of the visitor. The website www.gov.uk gives detailed and up to date information about requirements for specific countries and for regions of the UK.

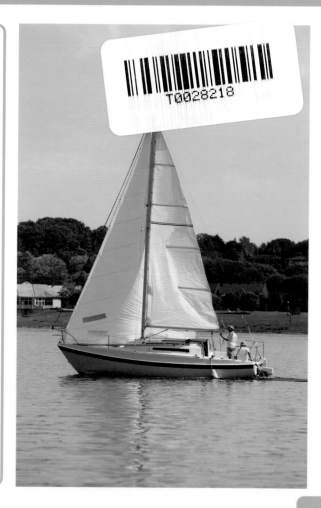

Contents

First Aid Protocol

- During any major incident involving injury or illness, the safety of the crew and vessel must remain paramount. The following sequence may help you to prioritise what to do while still providing first aid to the casualty. Continually reassess the ongoing safety. It may help to make brief notes if communication with external agencies is likely.

AVOID DANGER – TAKE CONTROL

1 Boat safety
2 Beware of hazards, e.g. electrics, rigging, carbon monoxide
3 Delegate if possible
   a sailing
   b first aid
   c communication
4 Clip on – first aider and casualty

INITIAL ASSESSMENT – PRIMARY SURVEY

1 **Ask:** Are you all right?
   Gently shake shoulders.

   AVPU
- Is the person **A**LERT?
- Is the person responding to **VE**RBAL enquiry?
- Is the person responding to **P**AIN?
- Is the person completely **U**NRESPONSIVE?

2 Consider mechanism of injury or illness.
   CONTROL CATASTROPHIC BLEEDING
   with direct or indirect pressure (see page 9).
   If **RESPONSIVE** – Provide appropriate first aid.
   If **UNRESPONSIVE** – Turn victim on to back, check **ABC** (see pages 6–8).
   A – AIRWAY
   B – BREATHING
   C – CIRCULATION

REASSESSMENT – SECONDARY SURVEY

1 **Full examination** (see page 31)
2 **Full history** past illness, medication, allergies
3 **Progress** of current condition
4 **SEEK HELP** (see pages 29–30)

DECISION

1 **Emergency** to save life or limb (see page 28) – Evacuation
2 **Urgent** Sail to nearest port immediately
3 **Expedite** Sail to convenient port
4 **Condition under control** Sail on

Basic Life Support – Resuscitation

- The guidelines for Basic Life Support (BLS) should be followed for any collapsed or unconscious person. If possible, delegate one crew member to read these instructions out loud while another member attends to the victim.

Possible causes of collapse

- Accident (e.g. immersion, electrocution)
- Injury (e.g. severe bleeding, head injury)
- Asphyxia (e.g. choking, smoke inhalation)
- Illness (e.g. heart attack, stroke, diabetes)
- Poisoning (e.g. stings, carbon monoxide)
- Anaphylaxis (e.g. severe allergy)

■ Avoid danger – take control

❶ Boat safety
❷ Beware of hazards
   e.g. electrics, rigging, carbon monoxide
❸ Delegate if possible
   - **a** sailing
   - **b** first aid
   - **c** communication
❹ Clip on – first aider and casualty

ASSESS RESPONSE

Ask: 'Are you all right?'

Gently shake shoulders.

AVPU (see page 31)

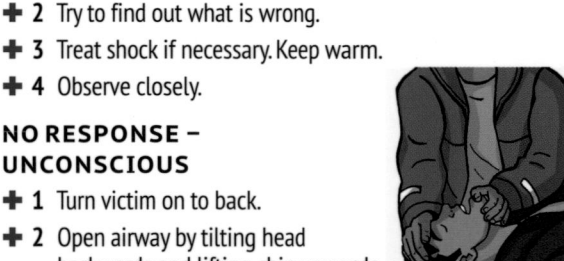

RESPONSE – CONSCIOUS

If patient responds and is **CONSCIOUS** with **NORMAL BREATHING**:

✚ 1 Ensure that victim is as safe as possible.
✚ 2 Try to find out what is wrong.
✚ 3 Treat shock if necessary. Keep warm.
✚ 4 Observe closely.

NO RESPONSE – UNCONSCIOUS

✚ 1 Turn victim on to back.
✚ 2 Open airway by tilting head backwards and lifting chin upwards.

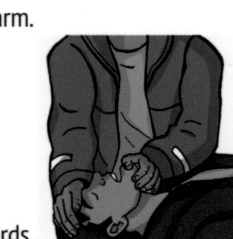

CHECK BREATHING

Caution: Just look if victim is not known or could have Covid-19.

Take only 10 seconds.

LOOK – for chest movement

LISTEN – at mouth for breath sounds

FEEL – air on your cheek

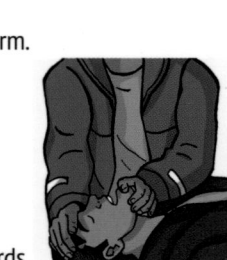

NORMAL BREATHING

✚ 1 Recovery position (see below).
✚ 2 Ensure that victim is as safe as possible.
✚ 3 Try to find out what is wrong.
✚ 4 Observe closely. Keep warm.

BREATHING IS OBSTRUCTED

If foreign object is suspected, treat for choking (see pages 11 and 12).

BREATHING ABSENT

Commence chest compression (see page 7).

RECOVERY POSITION

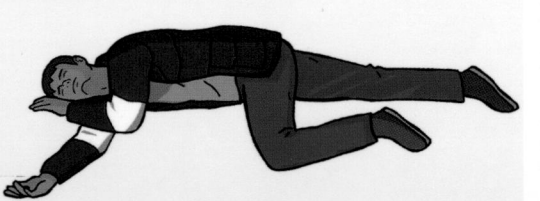

An unconscious breathing patient should be placed in the recovery position. The upper arm and leg are bent in order to prevent the casualty rolling on to his back or front. This position should allow breathing to continue unobstructed. It may be necessary to extend the neck and pull the chin forward if breathing appears obstructed. If possible turn patient on to other side every 30 minutes to relieve pressure on lower arm.

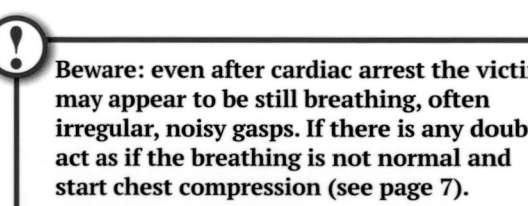

(!) Beware: even after cardiac arrest the victim may appear to be still breathing, often irregular, noisy gasps. If there is any doubt, act as if the breathing is not normal and start chest compression (see page 7).

Basic Life Support – Chest Compression

- If there is any doubt about the victim's Covid-19 status place a towel or cloth over the victim's nose and mouth. Perform chest compression only. Do not attempt rescue breathing.

Victim not breathing normally

❶ Start chest compression immediately.

❷ **DO NOT** even try to check for a pulse.

Chest compression

- Exert pressure only upon the centre of the breastbone (sternum) during compression.
- Compress the breastbone 5–6 cm (2–2.5 inches).
- Rate 100–120 per minute.
- **DO NOT** lift hands off between compressions.
- Press hard and fast. **DO NOT** stop.

Infants and children: Reduce the force of compression. Same rate of 100–120 per minute. Use 2 fingers for a baby and 1 hand for a young child.

At sea: External chest compression will be very difficult in a rolling, pitching boat and virtually impossible in a life raft. Try to lay the casualty on a firm surface.

■ Automated External Defibrillators

Automated External Defibrillators (AED) are designed to be used to treat cardiac arrest in a non-medical environment. There might be a rationale for providing this equipment in larger boats where a **dry** environment can be guaranteed or if crew/guests have known cardiac conditions. Crew should receive training.

- Switch on the machine.
- Attach pads to victim's chest.
- Follow the 'spoken' instructions from the machine.

Note: The environment, the victim and operator must all be DRY.

CHEST COMPRESSION

Step 1

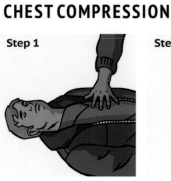

Lay the patient on a hard surface; kneel beside him; locate centre of breastbone.

Step 2

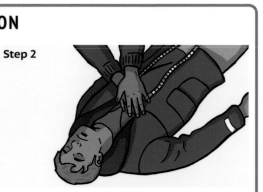

Place the heel of one hand on centre of victim's breastbone (sternum). Place the other hand on top and interlock fingers. Keeping arms vertical, compress 5–6 cm (2–2.5 inches) then release. Complete 30 compressions at a rate of 100–120 times per minute, then give 2 rescue breaths.

Step 3 for <u>one</u> operator

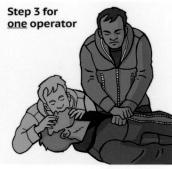

Continue chest compressions at 100–120 per minute; after every 30 compressions give 2 effective rescue breaths.

Step 3 for <u>two</u> operators

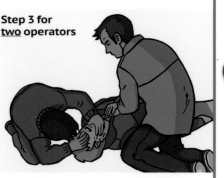

Continue chest compressions at 100–120 per minute; after every 30 compressions give 2 effective rescue breaths. Change tasks to prevent fatigue.

CHILD PATIENT

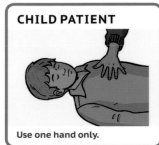

Use one hand only.

! DROWNING VICTIMS AND CHILDREN

Start with 5 rescue breaths (see page 8) before chest compression.

!

If you are unable or unwilling to give rescue breaths, continue chest compression at 100–120 per minute.

Basic Life Support – Rescue Breathing

- If there is any doubt about the victim's Covid-19 status place a towel or cloth over the victim's nose and mouth. Perform chest compression only. Do not attempt rescue breathing.

Rescue breathing

After 30 chest compressions (see page 7), open airway, tilt head, lift chin and pinch nose. Take in a normal breath yourself then blow steadily into victim's mouth. Watch for the chest to rise and fall – **look**, **listen** and **feel**.

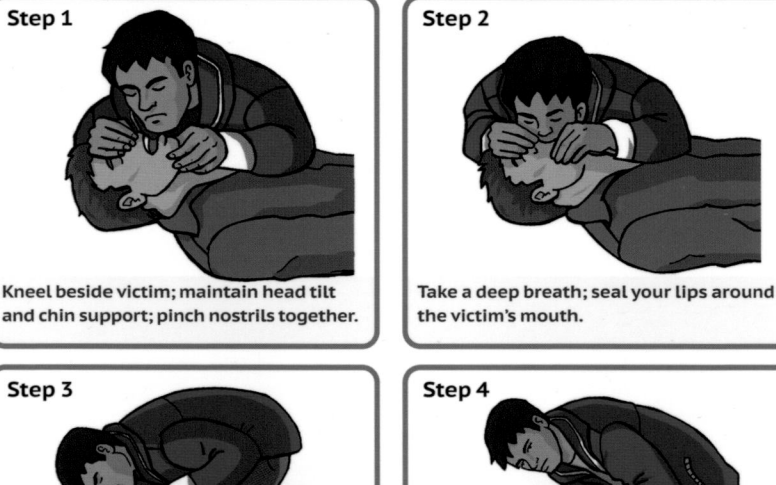

Step 1

Kneel beside victim; maintain head tilt and chin support; pinch nostrils together.

Step 2

Take a deep breath; seal your lips around the victim's mouth.

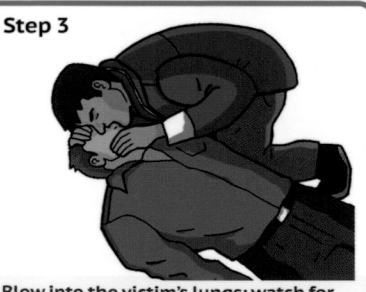

Step 3

Blow into the victim's lungs; watch for chest expansion. If expansion does not occur, adjust the chin support and tilt head further backward (see Step 1).

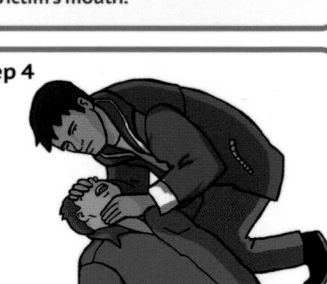

Step 4

Remove mouth; watch chest fall; repeat procedure. Give 2 breaths then return to chest compression at ratio of 30 compressions to 2 breaths.

MOUTH TO NOSE VENTILATION

May be used if the victim's mouth/jaw is seriously injured or if the victim is still in the water.

CHILDREN

DO NOT delay resuscitation in children for fear of causing harm.

- Give 5 rescue breaths before starting chest compressions and then continue CPR cycle using the same 30:2 sequence as for adults.
- Chest compression to at least $1/3$ depth of chest – use 2 fingers if infant is under one year; use 1 or 2 hands for a child.
- Check for signs of life – movement, coughing, breathing.
- Check for pulse for no more than 10 seconds.

DROWNING – ADULTS AND CHILDREN

Give 5 rescue breaths before starting chest compressions and CPR cycle (see page 14).

CPR – Cardiopulmonary Resuscitation

CPR is a combination of chest compression and rescue breathing.

1 Continue chest compression and rescue breaths at ratio 30:2.

DO NOT stop or interrupt CPR cycle 30:2 unless victim starts to breathe normally. **DO NOT** stop to check for pulse or breathing.

2 If rescue breaths do not make chest rise and fall then check mouth for obstruction and remove e.g. teeth, blood.

3 If two crew are available then swap round every 2 minutes to prevent fatigue. Minimise delay during changeover.

4 If you are unable or unwilling to give rescue breaths, continue with chest compressions only at a rate of 100–120 per minute.

5 Continue CPR until:
- Victim starts breathing (put him or her in recovery position, protect airway, treat shock, observe closely).
- You become exhausted or 30 minutes have passed.
- The safety of the boat and other crew is at risk.
- You have attempted re-warming a hypothermic victim who is still not breathing.

Bleeding & Shock

- Blood transports oxygen around the body.
- Without oxygen the vital organs such as the brain, heart, liver and kidneys cease to function.
- Loss of 25% of the body's blood can lead to death.
- A 70 kg (150 lb) man has 5 litres (8 pints) of blood.

CATASTROPHIC BLEEDING

TREATMENT

✚ Control life-threatening bleeding immediately with direct or indirect pressure.

✚ Apply a tourniquet for uncontrollable bleeding from a limb. Tightly applied bandage or strips of T-shirt or equivalent wrapped around the limb above the injury – tight enough to be very uncomfortable AND stop the bleeding.

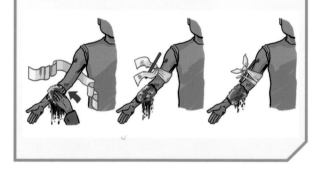

(!) **Ideally protective gloves should always be worn when dealing with blood or any body fluids.**

External bleeding

Bleeding can occur from any wound. In most cuts or wounds the blood oozes from the smallest blood vessels (capillaries) only, but in deeper cuts the larger vessels (arteries and veins) may be cut and the bleeding is more dramatic. Arterial bleeding produces spurts of bright red blood and is the most serious problem.

Treatment

❶ If possible check for foreign objects in the wound. Wipe or rinse off any small objects from the wound's surface using antiseptic solution or clean fresh water.

❷ Apply firm continuous direct pressure over the site of bleeding for at least 10 minutes. Use hand or fingers initially; substitute dressing pad when available and bandage firmly; if bleeding continues, add further dressing pads on top of initial pad. **DO NOT** remove the existing dressing as this may disturb any blood clot that has formed.

DO NOT bandage too tightly as doing so risks cutting off circulation to limb below wound.

❸ Elevate if bleeding is from a limb.

❹ Treat for shock (page 10).

❺ **DO NOT** apply a tourniquet unless there is uncontrollable bleeding which puts the person's life at risk. Note the time of applying the tourniquet. The survival of the whole limb is threatened by a tourniquet.

■ Nose bleed

May appear very dramatic. Control by sitting forwards and firmly pinching the soft part of the nose for a minimum of 15 minutes to allow the blood to clot. Loosen clothing at neck. **DO NOT** remove the pressure before 15 minutes. **DO NOT** blow the nose. If the bleeding continues, repeat the pinching for another 15 minutes or as long as necessary. Seek help if bleeding persists after 30 minutes of pressure.

BLEEDING FROM THE PALM

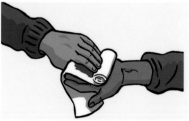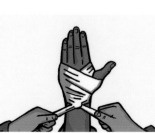

Apply pressure by bandaging a roll of gauze or a clean handkerchief into the palm.

Once the bandage is securely tied, the injured arm should be elevated.

NOSE BLEED

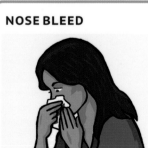

Lean forward and pinch the soft part of the nose for 15 minutes.

Bleeding & Shock

Internal bleeding

This is a difficult problem to manage at sea. The bleeding may not be obvious for some time and simple first aid is of limited use.

■ Possible causes:

- Fractures such as thigh bone or pelvis
- Crush injury of limb
- Penetrating injury, e.g. stab wound
- Blow to abdomen or chest, e.g. ruptured spleen
- Bleeding from stomach or bowel

Treatment

Treat for shock. **Emergency**; **evacuation**.

> ! **Ideally protective gloves should always be worn when dealing with blood or any body fluids.**

Shock

■ Possible causes include:

- Blood loss – internal or external bleeding
- Fluid loss – vomiting, diarrhoea, burns
- Heart failure – heart attack
- Severe infection – peritonitis, septicaemia (infection in the bloodstream)
- Anaphylaxis – severe allergy; peanut, bee sting
- Spinal cord injury

Treatment

❶ **BLS** – Basic Life Support (pages 6–8)

❷ Control bleeding

❸ Lay patient flat and elevate legs to 20 degrees after a faint, a minor injury or external blood loss

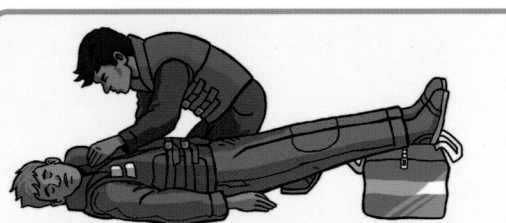

Exceptions to 3:
- Unconscious: use recovery position (page 6)
- Bleeding from mouth or face: use recovery position
- Chest injury or breathing difficulty: sitting sometimes preferred
- Heart attack, head injury

❹ Avoid movement; loosen tight clothes

❺ Keep warm. Provide reassurance

❻ Splint fractures

❼ Relieve pain; give strong painkillers
Exceptions to 7:
- confusion
- reduced consciousness
- breathing difficulty

❽ Give fluids if victim is conscious and able to swallow but not if there is internal bleeding or injury to chest or abdomen

---

IDENTIFYING A PATIENT WITH SHOCK OR INTERNAL BLEEDING

Rapid, weak pulse

Cold hands
– white or blue fingernails

Abdomen:
– may be rigid and tender if there is internal bleeding or organs are perforated

Rectal bleeding:
– blackish blood suggests bleeding from bowel
– bright red blood: probably piles

- Dizziness on sitting up
- Pale and sweaty
- Anxious or confused
- Thirsty
- Rapid breathing

Breathing Difficulty & Choking

- If insufficient air enters the lungs then insufficient oxygen reaches the vital organs and permanent damage or death will result.

Possible causes of breathing difficulty

! Asthma which does not respond to the patient's usual treatment is potentially very serious. *Urgent help is needed.*

■ Collapse
- Heart attack
- Stroke
- Head injury

■ Blocked airway
- Drowning
- Inhaled foreign body – choking
- Strangulation
- Vomit – unconscious or inebriated

ELECTROCUTION

Electric circuitry and lightning are causes of electrical injury at sea and ashore. Both may stop the heart and breathing, and both may cause deep burns.

1 Danger – turn off the power before touching the victim. **DO NOT** become a second casualty.
2 **BLS** – Basic Life Support (pages 6–8).
3 Recovery position if unconscious (page 6).
4 Treat burns. Treat shock.

■ Chest injury
- Rib fractures
- Damaged lung – pneumothorax

■ Inhalation of smoke or poisons
- Fire or exhaust fumes. If the boat is full of exhaust fumes then anyone below is inhaling carbon monoxide. This causes headache, drowsiness, unconsciousness then death.

■ Pre-existing lung disease
- Asthma (sufferers must carry **spare** inhaler & medication)

■ Paralysis or nerve injury
- Spinal cord injury
- Poisoning
- Electrocution (see panel)

Treatment
❶ Remove the cause if possible
❷ **BLS** – Basic Life Support (pages 6–8)
❸ Recovery position if unconscious (page 6)
❹ Loosen constrictive clothing.

Choking

Blockage of the airway by an inhaled foreign body is a common cause of death in otherwise fit persons. Peanuts are a frequent cause in children; lumps of meat in adults. (See illustrations of treatment methods on page 12.)

! **BREATHING DIFFICULTY –WORRYING FEATURES**

✚ **Breathing rate above 30 per minute**
✚ **Heart rate above 100 or below 50 per minute**
✚ **Core temperature above 39°C**
✚ **Shock – weak, thready pulse**
✚ **Reduced consciousness**
✚ **Exhaustion**

IDENTIFYING A PATIENT WITH BREATHING PROBLEMS

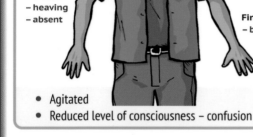

Mouth:
– froth
– blood

Lips:
– pale
– blue

Breathing:
– noisy
– wheezing

Coughing
Difficulty
speaking

Chest movement:
– rapid
– shallow
– heaving
– absent

Fingertips:
– blue

- Agitated
- Reduced level of consciousness – confusion

 DO Basic Life Support (pages 6–8)
Recovery position (page 6)
Control any bleeding

 DON'T Give priority to anything else

11

Breathing Difficulty & Choking

Choking

It is very important to recognise choking (airway obstruction by a foreign body). **DO NOT** confuse it with fainting, heart attack, seizure or other conditions that cause breathing difficulty and unconsciousness.

Choking usually occurs while eating: ask the victim 'Are you choking?'

■ Mild

Victim able to speak, cough and breathe.

Treatment
● Encourage to cough.

■ Severe

● Unable to speak (may nod and clutch neck).
● Unable to breathe or cough. May be unconscious.

Treatment, if conscious
● Alternate 5 back blows with 5 abdominal thrusts.

Treatment, if unconscious
❶ Open mouth and remove object if visible.
❷ Basic Life Support – begin CPR (see pages 6–8), starting with chest compressions.
❸ Even after recovery, help will be needed. Foreign material may remain in the air passages, leaving a persistent cough, difficulty swallowing or a sensation of something stuck in the throat.

Back blows × 5:

Lean victim forwards and support their chest with one hand. Give 5 sharp blows between shoulder blades with heel of hand. Check mouth after each blow.

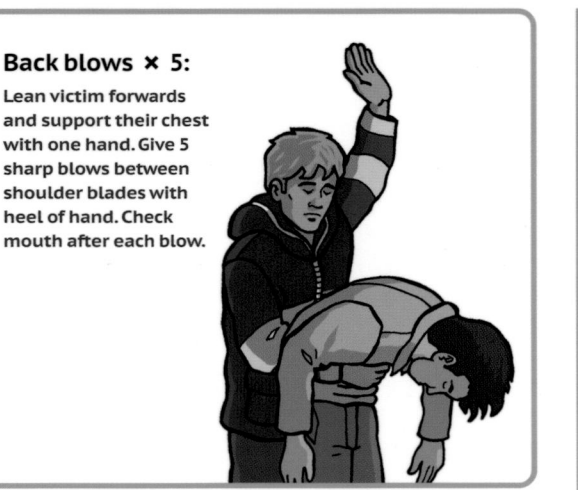

Abdominal thrusts × 5:

Arms around victim from behind. Put one hand in a fist just below breastbone and clasp fist with other hand. Thrust hands upwards into abdomen and compress lower chest so as to mimic coughing. Repeat 4 more times. Check mouth after each thrust.

INFANTS AND CHILDREN

If the infant or child is unconscious, open mouth and look for object. Single finger sweep **ONCE** only. **DO NOT** attempt blind or repeated finger sweeps – these can force the object further down the throat and airway.

INFANT:
✚ Perform 5 back blows with infant held head down.
✚ Chest thrusts rather than abdominal thrusts × 5 (firm thrusts in centre of breastbone).

CHILD OVER AGE 1:
✚ Perform 5 back blows with child's head down if possible.
✚ Abdominal thrusts × 5 (**DO NOT** do this for babies).

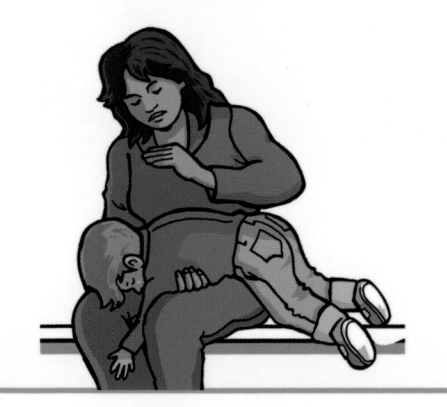

Burns & Scalds

Burns at sea can be caused by fire, electricity, chemicals and sun exposure. The principles of treatment are the same. Most burns will require specialist medical care ashore especially those greater than the area of the palm of a hand and where the skin has become white or charred. Burns to the face, hands, feet and genitals are of particular concern.

Breathing difficulty after smoke inhalation needs rapid assessment and treatment. Electrical burns might have little external visible damage but cause extensive internal harm. Major burns can cause shock as a result of the large loss of fluid through the burnt skin.

■ Rope burns

If severe, these require the same treatment as other burns.

DO Prevent sunburn
Keep burns clean
Drink plenty of water

DON'T Prick blisters
Apply ointments to broken skin

Treatment

❶ Stop the burning process without putting yourself at risk. Remove from smoke.

❷ **BLS** – Basic Life Support (pages 6–8) and treat shock.

❸ Remove any clothing or jewellery on or near the burn unless it is stuck to the burnt tissue.

❹ Cool the burn with cool or tepid water for 20 minutes – do not use ice. If water is in short supply immerse or douse the burnt area in seawater to cool down the tissue. Rinse with fresh water afterwards. Do not apply any oils or butter.

❺ Keep the victim warm – especially important in children where heat loss from the body is rapid.

❻ Loosely cover the burn in clingfilm or a clear polythene bag. **DO NOT** wrap anything around a limb – just cover the burn. Leave facial burns uncovered. Do not use fluffy dressings.

❼ **DO NOT** prick blisters. **DO NOT** remove loose skin.

❽ Treat pain with paracetamol and ibuprofen.

❾ Encourage oral fluids until passing a lot of urine.

❿ Sit patient upright if burn is on the head or neck to reduce swelling. Elevate burnt areas where possible.

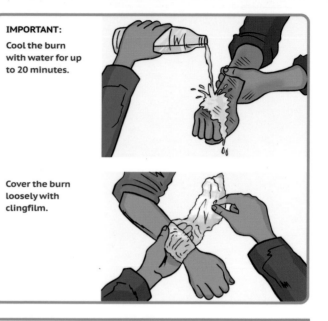

IMPORTANT:
Cool the burn with water for up to 20 minutes.

Cover the burn loosely with clingfilm.

SUNBURN

Sunburn is eminently preventable by the use of suitable clothing – including a wide-brimmed hat and sun-screen creams with a high protection factor (SPF 50). The cooling effect of the wind at sea often disguises the damage being done by the sun until too late. Crew with red hair or pale skin should take special care. **Sunburn at sea can be a serious problem and treatment is exactly the same as for other burns. DO NOT** prick blisters or rub ointment on broken skin.

Drowning & Hypothermia

Drowning

Resuscitation of an immersion victim at sea may be complicated by four factors:

❶ Injury or sudden illness may have caused the fall into the water in the first place.

❷ There may be a spinal injury (after diving accident or fall).

❸ Death due to heart failure or asphyxia may occur immediately on entering the water.

❹ Survival in the water will lead to hypothermia, which may cause unconsciousness without inhalation of water into the lungs. A crew member overboard wearing a lifejacket is at risk of hypothermia. A victim of hypothermia may appear pulseless and dead but full revival is possible.

Diving accidents

Any person who becomes unwell or unconscious after diving may have nitrogen decompression and/or air embolism. This can occur even after shallow dives, especially in inexperienced divers. Scuba equipment should only be used by trained divers.

Any unusual symptoms such as pain, weakness, numbness, strange behaviour or shortness of breath should be considered as a diving related injury.

Treatment – Diving accidents

❶ Immediate **BLS** – Basic Life Support (pages 6–8).

❷ Recovery position if breathing.

❸ Urgent help needed.

Note: avoid flying for 24 hours after diving.

Treatment – Drowning

❶ Danger – ensure that the rescuers are safe: **DO NOT** create a second victim.

❷ BLS: Basic Life Support (pages 6–8).
- Start with 5 rescue breaths before starting chest compressions and CPR cycle.
- **DO NOT** waste time trying to empty water from the victim's lungs.
- Regurgitation is very common. Turn victim on to side, clear mouth, turn on to back, resume CPR.

❸ Prevent cooling. Remove wet clothing and cover with dry sleeping bag or towels.

❹ Recovery position if breathing.

❺ Treat for shock. Horizontal or legs elevated. Delayed collapse is very common after immersion.

❻ Immersion victims will usually be cold and possibly unconscious. Although the victim may appear lifeless, full recovery is possible after rewarming. This may be difficult to achieve in a small yacht, but resuscitation and warming should be continued for as long as possible.

❼ Breathing problems can develop up to 72 hours after immersion. All immersion survivors who inhaled water should go to a hospital.

Hypothermia

Hypothermia may follow immersion (sudden) or prolonged (slow) exposure on deck. Symptoms include: shivering, irritability, lethargy, stumbling, slurred speech, loss of memory. The victim progressively develops cold, pale skin, slow breathing and a slow weak pulse, leading to collapse and unconsciousness. People who have drunk alcohol are particularly vulnerable to hypothermia.

Treatment

❶ Observe carefully for 60 seconds for any signs of breathing or other signs of life.

❷ If breathing:
- Put into recovery position (page 6) and commence re-warming.

❸ If no breathing and no signs of life:
- **BLS** as for drowning. Start with 5 rescue breaths then chest compressions and CPR cycle.

❹ Keep hypothermia victims horizontal; use gentle movement.

❺ Commence re-warming: replace wet clothing if possible and move out of the wind. Use sleeping bags, dry fleeces; warm with another crew member (buddy warming).

❻ Give hot sweet drinks if conscious.

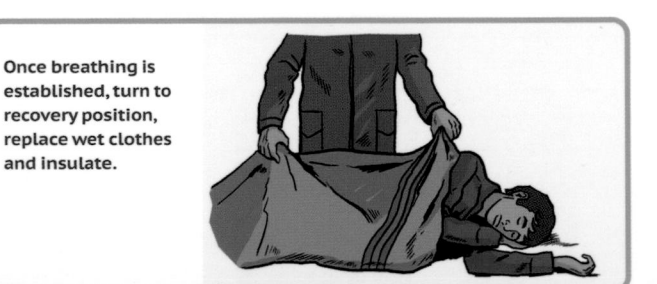

Once breathing is established, turn to recovery position, replace wet clothes and insulate.

Fractures & Sprains

Fractures and sprains can be caused by violent injury or fall.

Signs of fracture

- Pain
- Deformity
- Swelling
- Loss of movement
- Crepitus (grinding)

Complications of fractures

❶ Blood loss at the site of the fracture may be very significant and is most serious after fractures of the pelvis or thigh bone. In most bones it is initially apparent as swelling and then later as bruising. Internal blood loss may be sufficient to cause severe shock. Refer to shock on page 10.

❷ Interference with circulation of blood in limb due to swelling or bone deformity may cause the limb to be cold, pale, blue or numb. This is very serious.

❸ Damage to nerves can cause the limb to be very painful, tingling or numb. This is serious and can lead to permanent disability. Effective first aid can minimise the damage.

❹ Infection in compound fractures.

❺ In all cases specialist treatment should be sought as soon as possible in order to minimise the chance of long-term complications.

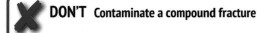 **DON'T** Contaminate a compound fracture

Treatment

❶ **BLS** – Basic Life Support (pages 6–8).

❷ Control external bleeding. Fractures (except those of the neck) **DO NOT** kill; bleeding does.

❸ Straighten limb, gently (where possible).

❹ Splint – improvise as necessary

❺ Elevate

❻ Treat pain

❼ Watch carefully for complications.

Splints

To be effective a splint has to prevent movement of the joints above and below the fractured bone. Padding is very important to prevent pressure damage. Bandages should not be so tight as to cut off the blood supply, especially as the limb will swell around the fracture. If the limb beyond the bandage or splint becomes painful or pale, it is essential to loosen the bandage before permanent damage occurs. Inflatable splints and malleable aluminium splints are useful. If evacuation is impossible for several days, bindings should be removed to assess the underlying skin for damage due to pressure or chafe. Try to clean the skin, while minimising any movement to the splinted limb.

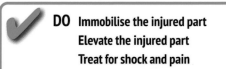 **DO** **Immobilise the injured part**
Elevate the injured part
Treat for shock and pain
Watch for complications

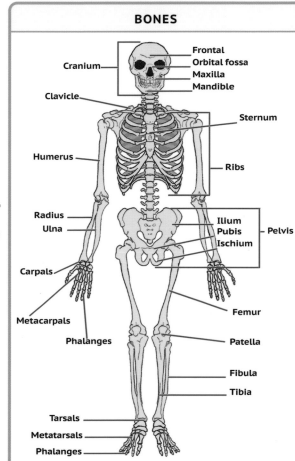

BONES

Frontal
Orbital fossa
Maxilla
Mandible
Cranium
Clavicle
Sternum
Humerus
Ribs
Radius
Ulna
Ilium
Pubis
Ischium
Pelvis
Carpals
Femur
Metacarpals
Phalanges
Patella
Fibula
Tibia
Tarsals
Metatarsals
Phalanges

Fractures & Sprains

Specific fractures

Ankle: An ankle fracture may be indistinguishable from a bad sprain. First aid treatment is the same for both. Immobilise in the neutral position with the foot at right angles to the leg. Rest and elevation of the leg are vital.

Back (spine): See neck.

Cheekbone: Requires specialist care but is rarely serious.

Clavicle (collar bone): Support the arm in a sling. (See Illustration 1.)

Compound fracture (broken bone pierces skin): Control bleeding. Clean with antiseptic solution, dress, splint, elevate, give antibiotics. **DO NOT** poke around at the site of a compound fracture – danger of infection. (See Illustration 2.)

Fingers and hand: Elevate and support, but in general leave unbandaged and encourage movement. A damaged finger may be splinted to an adjacent finger.

Foot and toes: Immobilise and elevate.

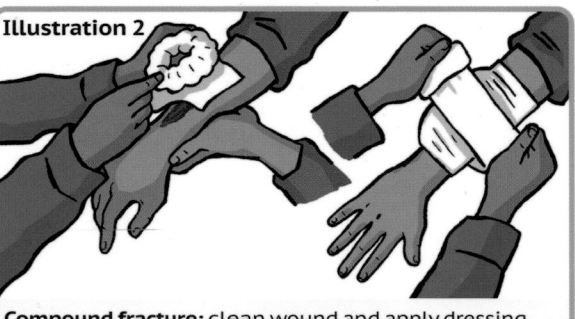

Compound fracture: clean wound and apply dressing.

Jaw (mandible): Beware of associated brain or spine injury. Remove blood and teeth fragments. Leave loose teeth in place. Maintain airway, bandage over head. Commence regular mouth rinses (e.g. antiseptic or salty water). Commence antibiotics. Only fluids by mouth.

Knee: The kneecap may be fractured by a violent direct blow. The ligaments or cartilages of the knee are often damaged by falls or twisting injuries. The knee may be very painful and swollen. Treat as for fracture. (See Illustration 4.)

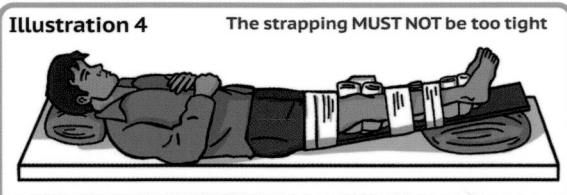

The strapping MUST NOT be too tight

Splint: for fracture of kneecap or lower leg.

Lower arm (radius and ulna): Splint, elevate, support in sling. **DO NOT** bandage too tightly. (See Illustration 3.)

Lower leg (tibia and fibula): Splint using generous padding and strap to the other leg with padding between the legs. (See Illustration 4.)

Nose: May cause bleeding or obstruct breathing through nose. Attempt to straighten immediately after the accident if possible. For bleeding nose, see page 9.

Pelvis: May follow major crush injury. **Serious and life threatening.** Treat shock and pain. **Emergency; evacuation.**

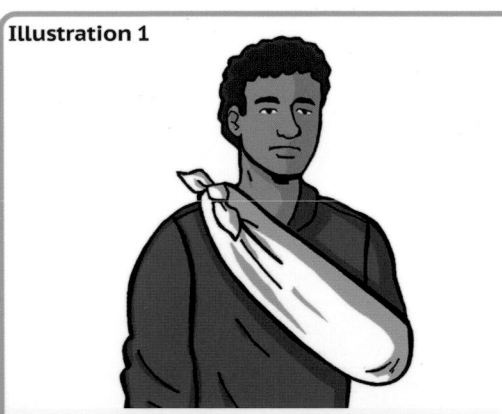

Arm sling: for fractures of clavicle (collar bone).

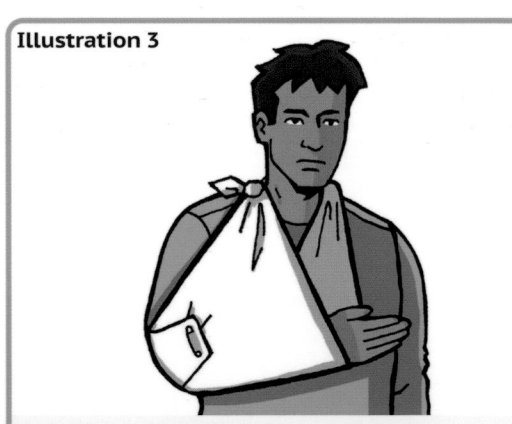

Arm sling: suitable for most arm fractures.

Fractures & Sprains

NECK AND SPINE INJURY

Spinal fracture may follow a fall, a direct blow or a violent whiplash-type injury. Damage to the spinal cord may occur at the time of the accident or, tragically, at a later time due to faulty handling of the casualty. You should have a high degree of suspicion and regard any neck injury as potentially serious.

A conscious patient may complain of pain, numbness, pins and needles, or weakness in arms and/or legs following spinal cord injury. **DO NOT** move unless essential.

For **neck injury** immobilise head and neck with rolled-up clothes or towels secured firmly on either side of head.

It is difficult to diagnose **spinal cord injury** in unconscious patients. Basic Life Support should still take precedence over any other first aid.

If necessary turn the unconscious patient into the recovery position (page 6) with smooth gentle movements, supporting the neck at all times.

Lift the patient as one rigid piece (log roll): **NEVER** allow the spine or neck to sag, twist or bend. **Urgent help is needed**.

If the accident occurs in port and breathing is adequate, then **DO NOT** move the patient until specialist help arrives.

Specific fractures *continued*

Ribs: Often very painful. Sit patient up, be aware of breathing difficulty, give painkillers. Bandaging or strapping is rarely helpful.

Shoulder injury: Often causes dislocation. If this has happened before, the patient may know what to do; otherwise treat as for fracture, but **DO NOT** attempt to correct the dislocation.

Skull: See head injury. **A potentially serious injury. Emergency; evacuation.**

Upper arm (humerus): Support the arm with a collar and cuff inside the shirt. Tie a clove hitch around the wrist and knot the ends of the bandage behind the neck. Then bind the limb to the chest with a large bandage.

Upper leg (femur): Considerable internal bleeding occurs. Treat for shock. Splint by strapping to other leg, **DO NOT** bandage too tightly. Extend splint above waist to prevent movement of hip. (See Illustration 5.)

Wrist: Refer to lower arm, page 16.

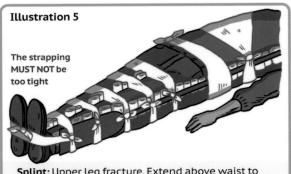

Illustration 5

The strapping MUST NOT be too tight

Splint: Upper leg fracture. Extend above waist to prevent movement

Strains and sprains

■ Back injury or strain

The person may have a history of previous back trouble or the injury may occur during awkward lifting. Treatment is initial rest (lie flat on a firm surface), painkillers and then gentle mobilisation. May need to rest for 24 hours or more. Leg weakness, numbness or bladder problems are serious complications.

■ Neck injury or strain

May follow lifting or twisting injury. Treatment is support (e.g. a towel around the neck), rest and painkillers. Tingling fingers, numbness or arm weakness are serious complications – obtain urgent medical advice. If in any doubt, immobilise and treat as for fracture. Faulty handling can cause paralysis.

■ Sprains

Any joint in the body can be damaged and the ligaments torn. The most commonly affected joints are shoulder, knee and ankle. The injury may be indistinguishable from a fracture and the first aid treatment is the same for both.

■ Strains and muscle injury

Can affect muscles or ligaments anywhere in the body. Muscle injury may result from a direct blow or strain (e.g. torn hamstring). Usually responds to simple treatment.

Treatment: **RICE**
- **R**est
- **I**ce (if possible at sea; avoid skin damage by ice).
- **C**ompression (firm bandage but not too tight).
- **E**levation
- Plus painkillers if needed.

Sudden Illness

Abdominal pain

Numerous possible causes. Important to identify the person who needs urgent medical attention. He/she will suffer more severe long-lasting pain that may be constant or occur in recurrent spasms. The pain may be localised or spread over whole abdomen. The abdomen will be tender when pressed and may be very rigid. The sufferer may also have fever, nausea and vomiting or generalised illness. He/she may develop shock. See page 10.

Treatment
Rest, treat shock, give pain relief, nothing to eat, sips of water only. Urgent help is needed.

■ Indigestion

Indigestion is a common cause of abdominal pain. The pain is usually restricted to the upper abdomen and may follow heavy alcohol intake and rich food. The abdomen is not tender or rigid.

Treatment
Frequent small sips of water, beware of dehydration, take antacid or omeprazole. Children are more liable to become severely dehydrated and should be encouraged to drink when ill.

Allergies

There is increased awareness about allergic reactions to foods, stings and medicines. Crew members with known allergies should alert other crew before sailing and avoid triggering agents (e.g. nuts, seafood). Known food triggers should probably be avoided for the whole crew.

Reactions can be mild (rash, redness, itchiness, wheezing, runny nose) and can be treated with antihistamine cream or tablets (e.g. chlorphenamine). Symptoms should settle once the allergic stimulus has been removed.

Anaphylaxis

Severe breathlessness, wheezing and/or collapse (anaphylaxis) is a medical emergency and requires full **BLS** – Basic Life Support (pages 6–8). Crew members with known severe allergies should carry at least two epinephrine (adrenaline) auto-injectors (e.g. Epipen) and one injection should be administered immediately once severe symptoms have developed. **DO NOT** delay administration.

Back pain

Back pain may develop following an accident, or heavy lifting, or for no apparent reason. There may be a history of previous back problems.

Treatment
Rest and painkillers. If there is numbness and weakness in the legs, or if bladder and bowel function are disturbed, seek help urgently.

Chest pain

May be caused by heart attack (see page 20), indigestion, oesophagitis, chest infection, fractured ribs, torn cartilage, or muscle strain.

Treatment
Painkillers – but avoid ibuprofen if indigestion is suspected. For indigestion and oesophagitis give medications such as omeprazole and Gaviscon.

> **(!)**
>
> **SIGNS OF POSSIBLE HEART ATTACK**
> + **Heart rate above 100 or below 50 per minute**
> + **Irregular heart beat or pulse**
> + **Weak, thready pulse**
> + **Breathing rate above 30 per minute**
> + **Reduced consciousness**
> + **Sweating**
> + **Vomiting**
> + **Pain spreading to jaw, arms or back**
> + **Known history of heart disease**

Sudden Illness

Constipation

Common problem at sea and even affects those who have no problems ashore. Poor diet, relative inactivity, dehydration and reluctance to use facilities are common causes. Crew members should be encouraged to drink water and soft drinks regularly and to eat fresh fruit and vegetables when available. Constipation lasting for a few days may contribute to the formation of piles (haemorrhoids) which may be painful and bleed. Special cream may alleviate the symptoms but will not treat the constipation.

Treatment
Rehydrate with non-alcoholic and caffeine-free drinks and take paracetamol or ibuprofen for pain. Take senna tablets if constipation persists.

Diabetes

Diabetics should not go to sea without taking adequate supplies of medication and instructing other crew in the management of potential problems. A diabetic may become unconscious if the sugar content in his blood is too high (insulin is needed) or too low (sugar is needed).

Treatment
If any doubt exists, it is advisable to give sugar first – sweets, soft drinks, pure sugar. Giving insulin inappropriately is dangerous. Urgent help is needed if recovery is not rapid.

Diarrhoea

Often follows some dietary indiscretion (food or water) but may be associated with other causes. In children in particular the amount of fluid lost from the body can be very serious.

Treatment
Encourage copious fluid intake (water with one teaspoon of salt and four teaspoons of sugar per litre); loperamide is a popular anti-diarrhoeal medication.

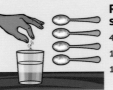

Rehydration solution

4 tsps sugar

1 tsp salt

1 litre water

Earache

Infection in the outer ear is common in hot climates and after swimming. The ear canal appears red and discharges.

Treatment
Painkillers. Clean the outer ear very gently and insert ear drops.

Infection in the middle ear may occur during a common cold. The pain is often severe and associated with fever and general illness. Eventually the ear drum may burst and release fluid trapped in the middle ear.

Treatment
Painkillers and antibiotics. Seek help if the pain increases. **NEVER** insert any object deep into the ear.

Epilepsy

Epileptics should not go to sea without taking adequate supplies of medication and informing other crew of potential problems. Most epileptic fits are self-limiting and should be treated by minimising damage to the body. The patient may fall to the deck or thrash arms and legs in an alarming manner, so try to protect him or her.

Treatment
Putting a piece of cloth between the teeth may reduce damage to the tongue. After a fit the patient may enter a deep sleep and should be placed in the recovery position while keeping a close watch on the airway. Seek help.

Eye problems

Many eye problems and injuries are potentially serious. Worrying symptoms include: pain, red eye, loss or blurring of vision, sensitivity to light and nausea. Urgent help needed. The victim may have a history of glaucoma. **DO NOT** use old or previously opened eye drops or ointments.

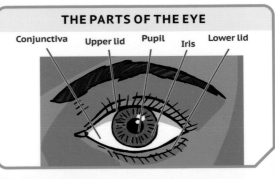

THE PARTS OF THE EYE

Conjunctiva   Upper lid   Pupil   Iris   Lower lid

■ Eye problems *continued*

Treatment – Infection

Superficial infection (conjunctivitis) produces a sticky, weeping eye. Treat with chloramphenicol ointment or drops applied 4 times per day. Seek help if rapid improvement does not occur. Dispose of the remaining drops or ointment once treatment is completed. Do NOT use again.

Treatment – Foreign body

If the object is imbedded in the eyeball, **DO NOT** attempt to remove it. Seek urgent help. Apply chloramphenicol ointment or drops; cover with pad.

Injury which results in pain, blurred vision or bleeding into the eye requires urgent help. Cover the eye with a pad.

For objects which are not imbedded, first flush the eye with clean water. Pull the bottom lid outwards while the victim looks up. Lift the object off the eye with the corner of a clean dressing or handkerchief.

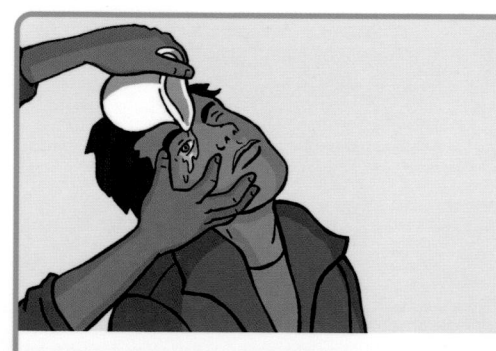

Flushing a foreign body from the eye.

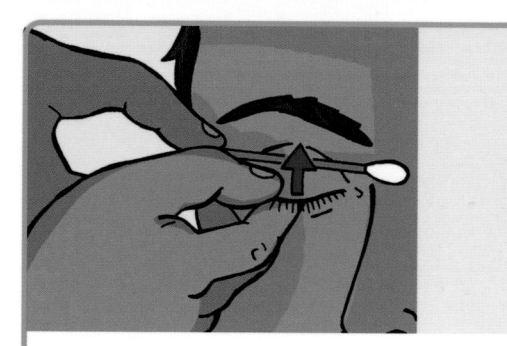

Inspecting under the upper lid.

To inspect under the upper lid, pull the lid outwards and then roll it upwards over something, e.g. a cotton bud. (See illustration above.) After removal, insert chloramphenicol ointment or drops and cover with a pad.

Treatment – Corrosive burns

Treat by flushing continuously with water for 15 minutes. Chloramphenicol ointment or drops. Eye pad. Painkillers. Urgent help is needed.

Fever

Normal body temperature is 36–37 degrees centigrade. Fever is always a sign of some underlying illness, with the common cold and throat infection being the most frequent causes. Infection anywhere in the body will produce raised temperature. When associated with abdominal pain, it may indicate something like appendicitis. In the tropics fever may mean malaria. In every case the underlying condition needs attention. The less serious cases should be treated with cool sponging, copious oral fluids, paracetamol and antibiotics if infection is obvious. Do not use antibiotics for common cold or upper respiratory tract infections.

Headache

Headache can be associated with seasickness and is commonly a result of dehydration. People feeling nauseous or unsteady will avoid moving and drinking, so dehydration is very common.

Those who suffer ashore with headaches, especially migraine, should bring their routine medication with them. Anxiety, motion sickness and dehydration can trigger a migraine attack.

Persistent severe headache associated with neck pain or stiffness, fever and blurring of vision is a medical emergency and requires specialist advice. Increasing headache following a blow to the head is potentially serious. Urgent help needed.

Heart attack

Severe crushing central chest pain, which may spread to neck or arm, accompanied by sweating, breathlessness and collapse. Any adult is at risk from the age of about 30 onwards. Rapid treatment will greatly increase chances of recovery.

Treatment

IMMEDIATE BLS – Basic Life Support (pages 6–8). Recovery position if unconscious (page 6). Close observation of pulse and breathing; strict rest, reassurance. Urgent help is needed. If available give one aspirin 300mg tablet immediately.

Sudden Illness

DAILY FLUID REQUIREMENTS
- Average sized man: 3.5 litres per day
- Average sized woman: 2.5 litres per day
- (From water, other drinks and food.)

Heatstroke

Heatstroke may follow exposure to high temperature with excessive fluid loss. Hot, red, dry skin, high temperature, rapid pulse, rapid breathing, fitting, collapse, unconsciousness. **DO NOT** underestimate potential seriousness.

Treatment

Get out of the sun; remove clothes; sponge down with cold water; drink copious fluids (water with one teaspoon of salt and four teaspoons of sugar per litre). Deterioration in consciousness is serious. **Emergency; evacuation.**

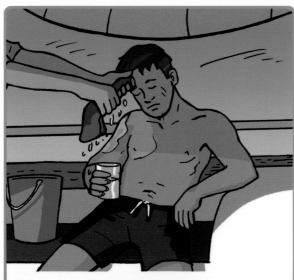

Keep cool in the shade, sponge down and give copious fluids.

Nausea and vomiting

Common causes at sea include seasickness, food poisoning and alcohol overdose. A variety of illnesses may start with nausea and vomiting, but the person will usually have other symptoms such as sore throat, abdominal pain or high temperature.

Treatment

Vomiting associated with continuing severe abdominal pain or vomiting of blood are serious problems for which urgent help is required. Other cases should be treated by avoiding food and taking frequent sips of water, and, if appropriate, indigestion tablets. See also seasickness (page 22).

Urinary problems

Pain in the lower abdomen or back associated with pain or difficulty passing urine (which might also be smelly) suggests a urinary tract infection. May cause fever and severe illness.

Treatment

Painkillers, copious non-alcoholic drinks and antibiotics. **May require evacuation**.

Sometimes with infection or injury passing urine becomes impossible (retention). Retention can also occur in the absence of infection in older men. It can only be treated by a trained person with a catheter and, if appropriate, consideration should be given to carrying a catheter on longer trips. **Urgent help required**.

Poisoning

Poisonous substances may be swallowed, or inhaled, or may penetrate the skin as in bites and stings (envenomation). Exhaust fumes, leaked bottled gas, and various industrial chemicals are toxic. The carbon monoxide in exhaust gas produces cherry lips and skin. Labels and containers often display advice on what to do in the event of poisoning and may suggest an antidote. Remember that many gases are heavier than air and will remain in the bilges despite adequate cabin ventilation. Pump out with bilge pump!

Treatment – General

❶ Ensure safety of first-aider and victim.
❷ BLS – Basic Life Support (pages 6–8).
❸ Recovery position if unconscious (page 6).
❹ Seek help early. In UK phone NHS 111.

Treatment – Bites and stings

Identify the cause if possible. Most bites only produce local pain and swelling, but some individuals may react severely and require full resuscitation. Before departure, anyone with known allergy to stings should seek advice from a doctor about provision of special injections (adrenaline) for an emergency.

Treat localised reactions with icepack or cool compress; antihistamines; painkillers; rest; elevation. In warmer waters highly deadly poisons are injected by marine animals such as sea snakes, jellyfish and octopuses.

Sudden Illness

Treatment – Bites and stings *continued*

Prevent drowning; avoid being bitten yourself during rescue; commence resuscitation and **DO NOT** stop (collapse may occur with alarming rapidity); pour vinegar on to jellyfish stings to prevent release of further poison. Wash any remaining tentacles off the skin with salt water. Bluebottle stings, sea urchin stings and some fish stings will be helped by immersing the affected area in hot water for up to 90 minutes. Non-tropical jellyfish stings require a cold pack for 10 minutes. Avoid movement of affected limb. Immobilise with a splint or sling. Starting at the fingers or toes, tightly wrap an elastic crepe bandage around the entire limb to delay the absorption of the poison. **DO NOT** use a tourniquet or cut into the site of the bite. **Emergency; evacuation.**

Treatment – Inhaled poisons
Move the victim into fresh air immediately and commence resuscitation if necessary. Strict rest afterwards. Serious breathing problems may develop afterwards and urgent help is needed.

Treatment – Swallowed poisons
DO NOT induce vomiting. Give copious fluids, e.g. as water, milk. Recovery position (page 6). Observe and seek help.

Seasickness

Disturbance of balance apparatus of body that may produce headache, lethargy, dizziness as well as nausea and vomiting. Motion is the prime cause, but the condition is aggravated by fear, anxiety, fatigue, cold, alcohol, strong tastes or smells and inactivity. The seasick crew may become pale, silent and inactive. There are often yawns or shivers.

The skipper should watch out for these signs, give encouragement, provide tasks on deck, and ensure that the crew member is wearing a life harness and is appropriately dressed for the conditions. Take food and fluid little and often; avoid alcohol and spicy or greasy food; keep warm and dry. If this fails, prolonged rest may be necessary. Intractable (incurable) vomiting becomes serious if it causes the victim to lose a large volume of body fluid.

Treatment
Up to 24 hours before going to sea start using anti-seasickness tablets or patches and avoid alcohol. Modern remedies are much less sedative and side effects such as dry mouth are less troublesome. Individuals vary as to which remedy suits them best.

Stroke

Sudden unconsciousness, paralysis or numbness often affecting one side of the body. Speech slurred and person disorientated.

Treatment
BLS, recovery position (page 6). Urgent help is needed, ideally within 3 hours.

Toothache

Treatment
If a hole is obvious, clean with a toothbrush and insert cotton wool soaked in oil of cloves. Give painkillers as necessary and antibiotics if the jaw becomes swollen. Fillings that fall out only warrant treatment if pain develops. Temporary filling kits are available for extended cruises.

Tooth socket – bleeding

Treatment
Bleeding may occur from the socket of a tooth that has been recently extracted or knocked out. Keep intact teeth for possible reimplantation by dentist. Treat by placing a piece of tightly folded gauze dressing or bandage over the socket and have casualty bite very firmly on it for 20 minutes or longer.

Unconsciousness & Head Injury

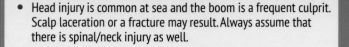

- Head injury is common at sea and the boom is a frequent culprit. Scalp laceration or a fracture may result. Always assume that there is spinal/neck injury as well.

For assessment of the unconscious person refer to the diagram in column 3. If breathing or pulse is absent commence **BLS** – see Resuscitation on page 6.

Possible causes of unconsciousness include: head injury, stroke, medical illness (e.g. diabetes), epilepsy, hypothermia, heatstroke, drug overdose (including 'social' drugs), alcohol, and electrocution.

Head injury

■ Head injury may cause:

❶ Immediate unconsciousness with rapid recovery. Concussion describes a temporary disturbance of brain function with a brief period of impaired consciousness following head injury. Following recovery there may be drowsiness, headache, dizziness and loss of memory for events surrounding the accident.

❷ Immediate unconsciousness with no recovery. **Very serious**.

❸ Delayed deterioration in a person who was initially conscious, or who was apparently recovering after being unconscious: increased drowsiness or headache, nausea and vomiting, double vision, confusion, convulsions, and eventually unconsciousness. **Very serious**.

> (!) **A fractured skull must be regarded as a very dangerous injury even if there is no apparent early disturbance of consciousness. Delayed deterioration occurs in many cases of skull fracture.**

Treatment

❶ **BLS** – Basic Life Support (pages 6–8).

❷ Recovery position if unconscious (page 6).

❸ Immobilise neck (see page 17).

❹ Control bleeding. Scalp wounds bleed profusely, but can be controlled with firm and sustained pressure.

❺ Then, according to degree of injury:

✚ **a** Immediate unconsciousness with rapid recovery.

Treatment: Recovery position if necessary; treat for shock. Observe very carefully for delayed deterioration. Seek advice; urgent.

✚ **b** Immediate unconsciousness with no recovery.

Treatment: Recovery position, maintain airway. Observe and record every 30 minutes: pulse rate, breathing rate, pupil size (both eyes); response to voice, painful pinch (AVPU). **Emergency; evacuation.**

✚ **c** Delayed deterioration.

Treat as for b above.

Emergency; evacuation.

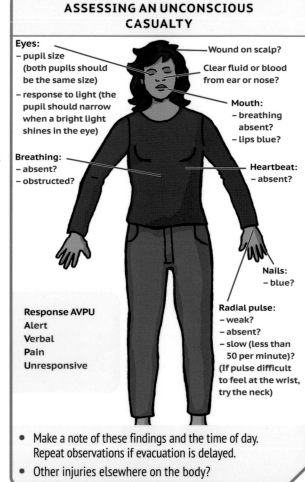

ASSESSING AN UNCONSCIOUS CASUALTY

Eyes:
– pupil size (both pupils should be the same size)
– response to light (the pupil should narrow when a bright light shines in the eye)

Breathing:
– absent?
– obstructed?

Response AVPU
Alert
Verbal
Pain
Unresponsive

Wound on scalp?

Clear fluid or blood from ear or nose?

Mouth:
– breathing absent?
– lips blue?

Heartbeat:
– absent?

Nails:
– blue?

Radial pulse:
– weak?
– absent?
– slow (less than 50 per minute)? (If pulse difficult to feel at the wrist, try the neck)

- Make a note of these findings and the time of day. Repeat observations if evacuation is delayed.
- Other injuries elsewhere on the body?

Wounds & Injuries

Abdominal injury

A blow to the abdomen or a fall that results in severe abdominal pain, shock or vomiting must be regarded as serious. There may be major internal bleeding.

Treatment
Treat for shock. Urgent help is needed.

Amputation

Bleeding is the main threat to life following accidental amputation of a limb or digit.

Treatment
Control catastrophic bleeding immediately using direct or indirect pressure. A tourniquet may be necessary. Treat for shock. Keep the severed appendage in a clean plastic bag. **DO NOT** store the limb in water. Severed limbs or digits can sometimes be reattached.

Bruises

Bruising is bleeding beneath the skin.

Treatment
Treat severe injuries with ice pack or cold compress, rest, elevation, painkillers.

Chest injuries

Serious chest injury usually results in fractured ribs, which are very painful and restrict breathing. The underlying lung may also be punctured or damaged. If a large number of ribs are fractured, or if there is a hole in the chest wall, the patient may experience extreme difficulty in breathing. This is a life-threatening condition. Shock may result from massive internal bleeding.

Treatment
❶ **BLS** – Basic Life Support (pages 6–8).
❷ Sit up if breathing is easier.
❸ Cover any wound that is bubbling or sucking air with a piece of plastic bag taped to the skin on three sides. This acts as a flap valve which allows air to escape but stops air entering the wound when the patient breathes in.
❹ Support painful chest wall with your hand. Avoid tight strapping or bandages that restrict breathing.
❺ Treat for shock. (See page 10.)
❻ Rest.
❼ Painkillers should be given.
❽ Observe closely for deterioration.
❾ Urgent help needed in all but simple cases.

Crush injuries

All or part of a limb may be crushed (e.g. between two boats), resulting in extensive bone and muscle damage. Delayed deterioration may occur.

Treatment
Control bleeding, treat shock, splint and elevate the limb, treat pain. Bleeding may be internal and concealed. Seek urgent help.

CUTS AND LACERATIONS

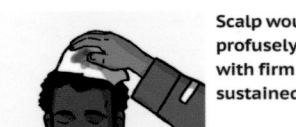

Scalp wounds bleed profusely. Control with firm and sustained pressure.

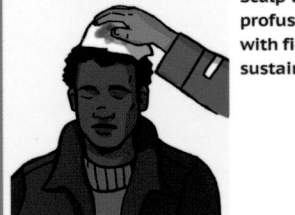

Closure of a laceration using adhesive suture strips.

Cuts and lacerations

Very common at sea. Often avoidable by paying attention to wire rigging and sharp edges. Prevention is better than cure.

Treatment
Control bleeding. Clean thoroughly with antiseptic. Remove dirt or other foreign objects.

✚ **a** Small clean cuts: Dry surrounding skin, then close using adhesive strips. (See illustration below.) **DO NOT** attempt to close wounds that are dirty, contaminated or infected (redness and/or pus).

✚ **b** Large deep cuts with uneven edges may be difficult to close with adhesive strips. Apply a sterile dressing and seek help. **DO NOT** attempt to suture wounds at sea.

✚ **c** Dirty wounds or wounds containing dead tissue must be left open. Clean as well as possible and apply dressing.

> **!** **Ideally protective gloves should always be worn when dealing with blood or any body fluids.**

Wounds & Injuries

Fingers and toes

Blood may collect under the nail following a blow to a finger or toe.

Treatment
Release the blood and relieve the pain by piercing the nail with a red hot needle or paper clip.

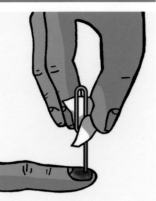

Blood under the fingernail: pierce the nail with a red hot paper clip or needle.

Fish hooks

Treatment
If the barb is embedded, then advance the hook until the barb exits through the skin, cut the barb off, and remove the hook.

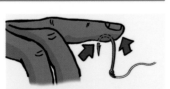

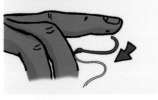

A method of removing a fishhook.

Skin problems

Treatments
Boil, carbuncle, abscess: DO NOT squeeze because this may spread the infection and make the problem worse. If temperature is high, give antibiotics. Hot compresses are sometimes useful. If a yellow head appears, it may be punctured with a sterile blade or needle to drain the pus.

Sores: Clean with disinfectant and keep as dry as possible. Apply antiseptic or antibiotic ointment.

Blisters: DO NOT prick blisters.

Cold injury – chilblains: Keep hands and feet warm and dry. Protect skin. Avoid infection.

Trench foot: Feet are painful, pale, cold, wet and swollen. Use warm, dry socks and loose, dry, breathable footwear.

Splinters

A common problem at sea; may be wood, fibreglass or metal. Infection is the main danger.

Treatment
Use a clean needle and tweezers to remove splinter if possible.

DO Control bleeding first
Clean thoroughly

DON'T Try amateur surgery
Close a dirty wound

HIV AND HEPATITIS

To avoid possible infection with HIV or hepatitis, medical and dental personnel wear protective gloves when in contact with a patient's body fluids (blood, saliva, tears, urine, faeces, etc.). First-aiders should take the same precautions, although life-saving treatment should never be delayed because gloves are not available.

Disposable examination gloves are readily purchased and should be thrown away (not overboard) after single use.

First Aid Kit

Any boat, other than a small dinghy, should carry a first aid kit. The contents of the kit will depend upon the intended sailing distance, the number of crew and the first aid expertise available onboard.

The suggested list of items on page 27 would make up a suitable first aid kit for coastal cruising or racing offshore. Smaller vessels or day sailors may manage with fewer items, but only if they are not far from help ashore.

A vessel may seem to be close inshore, but in fact may be some time away from skilled medical assistance should it be needed. Bandages and dressings to control bleeding or immobilise a fracture should therefore be considered essential.

- The first aid kit should be stowed in a container that is waterproof, crushproof, lightweight and clearly marked. A plastic food container may be suitable.
- It should be clearly marked and the crew must know where the kit is stored.
- The contents should be checked prior to each cruise and replenished as necessary. Many drugs become out of date and should be replaced as necessary.
- Ready-made kits are available but a home-assembled kit is cheaper and can be tailored to suit personal needs.

A grab bag with basic first aid kit should be available to take to a life raft.

Prescription items

Some items in the list require a doctor's prescription. Your pharmacist or doctor will advise when this is necessary and may also suggest alternative medication, especially for antibiotics. New versions of medication appear regularly.

Individual crew medication

- Any crew member who takes regular medication must bring sufficient supplies to last the whole voyage. Replenishment may not be possible without a prescription or when abroad.
- The skipper must be aware of any crew member who has a chronic illness such as asthma or diabetes.
- The skipper must be aware of any crew members with known anaphylaxis. The crew member must bring at least two epinephrine (adrenaline) auto-injectors (e.g. Epipen).

PREPARATION, PLANNING, PRECAUTIONS

Before departing on extended cruising consider the following:

- **Pre-existing conditions** (e.g. diabetes, asthma, heart disease, epilepsy).
- **Medication** – crew must bring their own special medication.
- **Immunisation** – see Department of Health's 'Advice for Travellers'.
- Dental check-up.
- **First aid kit**.
- **Advanced first aid training**.
- **Medical insurance** – UK Global Health Insurance Card.
- **Communication**. Identify radio procedures before departure.

- People who are susceptible to seasickness should bring their own preferred remedies.

Extended cruising or ocean racing

Anyone planning a blue-water passage or long-distance cruise will need to give special thought to the medical kit. Experienced advice should be sought regarding the items they should carry.

Even simple medical items may be hard to find or expensive when abroad and a good stock of basics should be carried. More advanced medication may be totally unavailable. Medical assistance may be hard to obtain, especially in the tropics or in areas where other special problems such as malaria exist.

A full course of vaccinations and malaria prevention may need to commence some months prior to departure. Specialised travel clinics will help, and in the UK the Department of Health provides 'Health Advice for Travellers'. Most GP surgeries will also be able to advise on specific health requirements for different parts of the world. There is a good selection of websites giving health advice for travellers. Check that the information is up to date because advice can change from week to week.

> **(!)** Extended cruising requires that at least one person aboard should have advanced first aid training and understand the correct use of the more detailed medical kit that is likely to be carried.

First Aid Kit

First aid training

A basic knowledge of first aid is especially important for seafarers. There are many instances involving, for example, drowning or choking where instant action is needed and there is no time to 'stop and read the book'. While this book gives instructions in dealing with most common emergencies, formal training is extremely worthwhile. In Great Britain training courses are organised by the RYA, the British Red Cross Society, St John Ambulance and many local yacht clubs.

Recommended basic first aid kit

Note: In addition to the main kit it is useful to keep a more accessible small kit containing items such as adhesive plasters, seasickness tablets, sunblock cream etc. Store this in the heads or galley and keep the main kit sealed for more serious occasions.

- Alcohol swabs
- Assorted adhesive plasters
- Adhesive elastic strapping 75 mm × 1
- Adhesive suture strips (e.g. Steristrips™)
- Adhesive waterproof strapping
- Cotton bandages 50mm × 2
- Cotton buds
- Cotton wool
- Crepe bandage 75 mm × 2
- Disinfectant solution (antiseptic)
- Disposable gloves
- Eye pad
- Finger bandage
- Forceps
- Gloves
- Hand sanitiser
- Paraffin gauze sterile dressings
- Petroleum jelly
- Safety pins
- Scissors
- Splints
- Sterile non-adhesive dressing
- Thermometer
- Triangular bandage × 2
- Tweezers
- Wound dressings (1 large, 1 medium)

AILMENT/USE	GENERIC DRUG NAME	DOSAGE
Allergies	Chlorphenamine	4mg every 4–6 hours. Max 24mg / 24 hours
Antibiotics	Co-amoxiclav*	600mg every 6 hours
	Azithromycin	500mg once daily for 3 days
	Doxycycline	200mg on first day, then 100mg daily
Athlete's foot	Miconazole	Apply twice daily
Chafed or dry skin	Moisture cream	Apply as often as necessary
Constipation	Senna tablets	2–4 tablets per day
Diarrhoea	Loperamide	2 capsules initially then 1 at each loose stool
Ear infection (external)	Corticosteroid/antibiotic drops	Apply every 6 hours
Eye infection	Chloramphenicol ointment or drops	Apply every 3–4 hours
Indigestion	Omeprazole	20mg twice daily
	Gaviscon	10–20ml after meals
Pain relief	Ibuprofen**	400mg every 8 hours, after food
	Paracetamol	1g every 6 hours
	Dihydrocodeine	1–2 tablet(s) (30mg) up to 6 hourly
Seasickness	Cinnarizine (Stugeron)	2 tablets 2 hrs before travel then 1 every 8 hours
	Hyoscine patches	Apply behind ear 5 to 6 hours before sailing. Apply new patch after 3 days if necessary.
Skin infection	Fucidin ointment	
Stings & itches	Calamine lotion	
Sunscreen	Waterproof sunscreen SPF 50+	
Toothache	Oil of cloves	

* Anyone allergic to penicillin should not take Co-amoxiclav.
**Ibuprofen should not be given to asthmatics or anyone with stomach ulcers or allergy to aspirin-type drugs.

• For more detail on all aspects of rescue see:
www.rya.org.uk/knowledge-advice

Man overboard

It is vital to prevent this happening in the first place.

Ideally safety harnesses and lifejackets should be worn by all crew on deck at all times, but should be mandatory at night, in rough weather, or outside the cockpit. Only non-slip deck shoes and boots should be worn.

■ Retrieval of a man overboard

There are several methods for retrieving a man overboard. In any boat the most effective drill will depend on the crew size and strength, as well as on the type of boat and the gear carried.

The problem is not only in getting a lifebuoy to the man and bringing him back alongside the boat but also in hoisting him aboard. This is particularly difficult with a small number of crew. It is vital that an individual is nominated to keep sight of the victim at all times.

All skippers must think about this and work out the most effective drill with the normal crew in the boat before it happens. It is important that this whole scenario should be rehearsed by every yacht crew using their chosen equipment and technique. Low transoms and swim platforms will help in some vessels.

■ Suggestions

If conditions make close manoeuvring difficult, then an appropriately attired crew member attached to a light floating line can bring the casualty alongside the vessel.

A halyard can then be attached to the victim's safety harness, or to a rope strop tied around the chest and under the arms, to winch the victim out of the water. It may also be possible to hoist a victim into a dinghy or life raft alongside.

Several devices are available to help with the difficult manoeuvre of getting a casualty back on board. All these devices should be tested in a calm situation before they are needed in earnest.

■ Once aboard

Perform immediate assessment and commence resuscitation on deck if necessary; **BLS** – Basic Life Support (pages 6–8). Only then consider removal below deck. For subsequent management see pages 6 and 14.

> **!**
>
> **REMEMBER**
> + **The victim may be cold, weak and frightened.**
> + **The victim may be unconscious.**
> + **The victim may have swallowed or inhaled a large quantity of sea water.**
> + **A wet fully clothed body, unable to cooperate, is both heavy and awkward.**

Helicopter evacuation

If helicopter evacuation is necessary, then careful preparation will ensure safe transfer of the casualty. Keep the casualty warm and dry. Dress him in oilskins. He must carry a waterproof wallet containing:

❶ Identification (passport if necessary)

❷ Details of next of kin

❸ Medical checklist (see page 31)

❹ Money and/or credit card

❺ Mobile phone

The mast and rigging are hazardous to the helicopter. Evacuation of a casualty is normally undertaken by means of a high-line transfer. Any lines dropped by the helicopter should be allowed to dip in the sea before being grabbed by the yacht crew to avoid static electricity shock. **NEVER** secure the helicopter line to the boat at any time.

The yacht will be instructed via VHF by the helicopter crew to sail close to the wind on port tack or motor head to wind. Smaller boats may be asked to remain stationary. All unused sails and loose objects should be secured. Once the helicopter is hovering it will be almost impossible to communicate because of noise. Pilots will give clear instructions during their approach.

A weighted line will be lowered into the cockpit and the yacht crew will be briefed to take in the slack. The winchman will then be lowered alongside the yacht and the helicopter crew will indicate when the yacht crew should pull him aboard.

Once on board, the winchman will take charge of evacuating the casualty by whatever means are appropriate after taking any immediate first aid steps. Tension should be kept on the high-line but it should never be secured to the boat during evacuation. The helmsman must steer a steady course at all times.

Communications

Emergency communications

Communications should be used to (1) obtain advice and/or (2) to seek assistance and evacuation of the casualty.

To obtain radio medical advice, contact HM Coastguard on **MF DSC**, **VHF DSC**, **VHF Channel 16** or **INMARSAT**. If HM Coastguard station cannot be raised, calls should be addressed to: **ALL STATIONS.**

In an emergency a mobile phone or satellite phone can be used, dialling 999 (UK: ask for coastguard) or 112 (international). This should not be the only means of making emergency communication on board.

Mobile phone signals in coastal waters have improved significantly and this may be the simplest and most secure way to communicate and obtain advice. If a good signal exists more extensive advice can be easily obtained from the NHS (UK) website www.nhs.uk. Scroll to the health A–Z section for a simple index.

Often in an emergency situation the radio may have to be operated by someone with no previous radio operating experience. Everyone who goes to sea should learn to operate the radio. Operating instructions for sending a distress message should be posted alongside the radio.

> **Help and advice can only be given if there is an accurate account of the patient's condition.**
>
> **Use the medical checklist on page 31 to ensure that the complete details are relayed.**

The urgency signal PAN PAN

RADIO DISTRESS SIGNAL PROCEDURE

1　**"PAN PAN"** (repeated × 3)

2　**Coastguard station name** (repeated × 3) **or "ALL STATIONS"** (repeated × 3)

3　**This is** ....
　　Yacht's name (repeated × 3)

4　**"Call sign and MMSI number"** ....

5　**"Number of people on board"**

6　**"In position"**

7　**"I require medical advice"**

8　**"Over"**

Please fill in information on dotted lines before voyage

The answering station will then direct the caller to a working frequency, where more details will be sought about the type of illness or injury and the nearest possible point of landing or helicopter assistance (if required). Callers may be redirected to a medical adviser.

PAN PAN is an internationally recognised distress call, and most European coast and radio stations can give advice in English. More details can be obtained from the Admiralty List of Radio Signals Vol 1 (NP 289), from Admiralty Maritime Communications (NP 289, NP 291), from **Reeds Nautical Almanac** and from some cruising guides.

Important information

TELEPHONE NUMBERS

Hospital	
Doctor	
Local Coastguard Operations Centre	
National Maritime Operations Centre	+44 2392 552100

VHF CHANNELS AVAILABLE ON BOARD

Channel	Use for

- For more detail about calling for help see: www.rya.org.uk/knowledge-advice

Communications

Distress signals

There are many instances when a vessel may be considered in distress. From a medical perspective, distress situations might occur when:

❶ A member of the crew is seriously ill or injured.

❷ A key member of a small crew is incapacitated so that the boat can no longer be sailed safely.

> **SOS**
>
>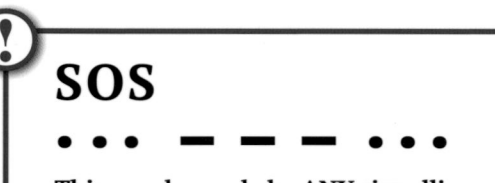
>
> This may be made by ANY signalling method and is readily understood. Use a mirror, torch, horn, whistle, etc.

> The role of flares has been significantly downgraded by the MCA (Maritime and Coastguard Agency). Red button DSC (Digital Selective Calling) for emergency communication and EPIRBs (Emergency Position Indicating Radio Beacon) are far more reliable, but flares may be the only thing available in some yachts.

■ Other signalling methods

Although radio is the most common method of calling for assistance, there are other types of distress signals available when radio communication cannot be made or when a radio is not carried. In these instances the following are recognised distress signals:

SOUND

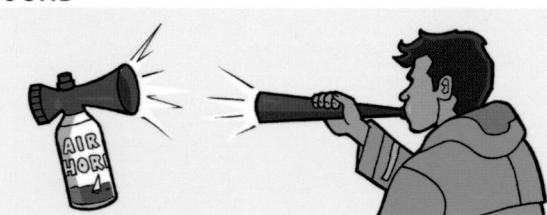

A continuous blast on a horn or a whistle is useful for attracting attention and is a recognised distress signal.

VISUAL

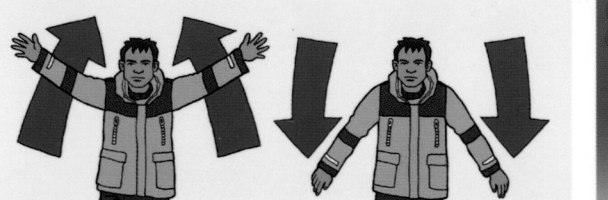

Raising and lowering arms slowly and repeatedly is a distress signal.

FLARES

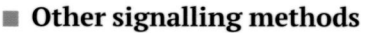

Red parachute flares are the most effective and can be used by day and by night.

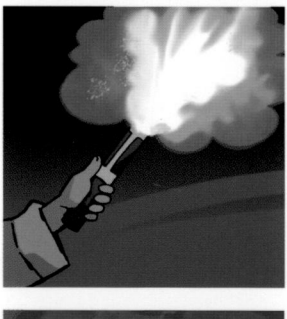
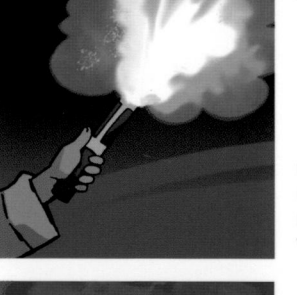

Red hand flares are shorter range, but are useful for pin-pointing your position at night when help is coming.

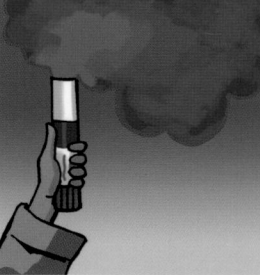

Orange smoke flares are used by day.